ARTHRITIS – the Conquest!

The basic cause of arthritis is self-poisoning resulting from faulty nutrition. But arthritis is *not* incurable and this book explains how early measures based on fasting, special diet, gentle exercise and water treatment, can restore mobility to diseased joints.

By the same author
DIETS TO HELP KIDNEY DISORDERS
DIETS TO HELP PROSTATE TROUBLES
DIETS TO HELP PSORIASIS

In this series
BANISHING BACKACHE AND DISC TROUBLES
HEADACHES AND MIGRAINE
NATURE CURE FOR PAINFUL JOINTS
NATURE CURE FOR PROSTATE TROUBLES
NATURE CURE FOR SHINGLES AND COLD SORES
SELF-TREATMENT FOR COLITIS
SELF-TREATMENT FOR HERNIA
SELF-TREATMENT FOR SKIN TROUBLES

ARTHRITIS
– the Conquest!

Harry Clements N.D., D.O.

THORSONS PUBLISHERS LIMITED
Wellingborough, Northamptonshire

First published as *Nature Cure for Arthritis* 1968
Second Impression 1970
Second Edition, revised and reset, 1973
Ninth Impression 1984

ISBN 0 7225 0216 8

Printed and bound in Great Britain
by Richard Clay (The Chaucer Press) Ltd.,
Bungay, Suffolk.

Contents

Foreword

AS THIS BOOK is intended to be a practical and self-help book no attempt has been made to go into details of the complaint discussed that would only complicate the issue for the ordinary person who wants to get well. The view is taken that arthritis is a condition of the body, where the joints are mainly involved but where the underlying condition of the system is the important factor upon which the sufferer must focus his attention. From these premises we argue that the individual can do a great deal for himself in overcoming his infirmities by centring his attention on the way in which he lives, and the various daily habits which he has developed. It follows that the impaired state of health from which he suffers is, in effect, the result of mistaken ways of selecting foods, of using them without discrimination in his diet, and thus undermining, by inadequate and faulty nutrition, the disease-resisting qualities of his body. We believe this is the fundamental problem that must be solved if we are to eradicate arthritis and the allied complaints.

The effects of arthritis, being centred upon the structures and functions of the joints, lead to an impairment of the body's mechanical efficiency, and this becomes a matter of great importance in managing the disease. The sufferer must learn not only how to manage the trouble from the nutritional and biochemical point of view but also to understand something about the mechanical principles of joints so that he can avoid unnecessary strain in their usage and thus prevent further spread and complications of the complaint. In this respect the individual must be called upon to play a conscious and responsible part in promoting effective treatment. Only he himself can attend to this essential matter that must become an integral part of his daily life.

For these reasons, self-help is of particular importance in the management of arthritis; and as it is abundantly clear that medicine at the present time can offer no solution, then the nature cure principles which we are propounding are surely worth a thorough trial.

Introduction

AS A GENERAL rule arthritis is regarded as being incurable, and one must say that if the condition is allowed to go on until radical changes have taken place in the joints and the tissues associated with them, full recovery may not be made. But such a statement is true of many diseases; if early stages are neglected then the body has to do the best job it can in the circumstances and permanent damage may be unavoidable. In all forms of disease — and this is especially true of arthritis — curability depends upon promptness in tackling the very first symptoms and on the effectiveness with which suitable treatment is applied. In this respect drug treatment is doubly dangerous: first of all, none of its advocates claim that it can cure arthritis; and secondly, by masking the symptoms and suppressing pain, it enables the disease to proceed unchecked.

We must be clear as to what we mean by the word cure. All forms of disease are not separate entities in themselves; they are processes involving the whole system, with changes occurring in all the body's tissues and functions. When we talk of a specific cure we imply that we can use a specific agent to change all this and to restore the whole system to normality. On the face of it this may seem possible — certainly it is desirable — but when we consider the many factors involved in a condition such as arthritis, then many doubts enter our minds. What we really do by the use of such agents is not to bring about a natural recovery from the disease reaction but to divert the reaction that is taking place. In short, we change the pattern of the disease without restoring the natural balance within the system. Therefore, the word cure, used to imply that an external agent can restore natural functions, has little meaning.

The idea that each disease needs a special agent to cure it has led to the fallacious notion of treating all forms of disease as distinct conditions bearing little relation to each other. Thus we have named some four hundred disease reactions which are thought of as different diseases, and this has given rise to the impression that each must be met with its own special agent in order to cure it. The main purpose served by this division of diseases is that when a new disease reaction arises — sometimes the result of treatment employed — no one thinks the remedy is to blame.

Many Forms of Arthritis
There are of course many forms of arthritis; indeed, one might almost say that each individual sufferer represents a different form of it, since no two individuals are completely alike or react to their environment in the same manner. Broadly speaking, the ordinary person thinks of two forms of the trouble: the rheumatoid kind and osteo-arthritis. The American Rheumatism Association divided the subject up into four groups: rheumatoid arthritis, of the peripheral joints and the spine; degenerative arthritis, which could be localized or generalized; fibrositis which also might be localized or generalized; and arthritis due to gout. Some investigators have suggested that there might be as many as fifty different kinds of arthritis, but for the ordinary person this simply magnifies the subject beyond common understanding.

Dividing the subject up in this way leads to the conclusion that if there are many forms of the disease then each must have its own remedy; the whole field then becomes endlessly complicated. Apart from the medical agents employed, there are many remedies that have been used to treat the trouble. One finds persons who are willing to declare that his or her arthritis has been cured in this way. As a rule all these so-called cures are based on the changes which nature brings about in the early stages of the disease-reaction. We should bear in mind that the *vis medicatrix naturae*, or the healing power of nature, is always operating in the body and spontaneous recoveries from all kinds of troubles may take place, including, as has been well established, such degenerative diseases as cancer. What we should try to do in such cases is to learn what the real factor is that brings about recovery and not delude ourselves with remedies that are akin to witchdoctoring.

The present obsession with finding cures for the various diseases, including of course arthritis, tends to do a great deal of harm since it fosters the idea that whatever may be the cause of the trouble is of relatively little importance. If a cure can be found, why bother about finding the causative factors? But cures do not work that way. Where can one think of a cure in the whole history of medicine that has wiped out a disease? If we think of the deficiency diseases that have been overcome it is due to the improvement in nutrition and the standard of living. And this is true of all the diseases that have disappeared. Treatments such as insulin and liver treatments did not abolish the disease; they perpetuated both the disease and the remedy.

Cortisone and Aspirin

The same thing might have happened with arthritis. Many people thought that the discovery of cortisone meant that, like diabetes, we should have a remedy for arthritis, usable not as a curative agent but as a constant form of treatment, employed regularly to maintain the necessary cortisone supply. In a word, we should have had a scheme for the perpetuation of the remedy and the disease. As events turned out, however, cortisone produced all kinds of serious side-effects and its use has now been largely abandoned. Aspirin, of course, has been the great pain-killer and arthritis remedy for many years, no doubt giving relief from some of the more acute symptoms but offering no promise of a real cure in the true sense of the term. Now after years of its use it has been found that aspirin can produce internal bleeding, and in the case of peptic ulcers may induce perforation and other dangerous conditions. One could go on listing all the other remedies — gold salts, and so on — that have had their day and are now carefully buried in the archives of medical history.

No doubt as long as we have a pharmaceutical industry and a medical profession obsessed with drug therapy as a method of treating disease, the search for a remedy, or for many remedies, for the different forms of arthritis will go on. The only alternative to this kind of thinking lies in the imperative need to pay more attention to finding the cause of disease rather than to search for cures. In the long run we must see that the only efficient answer to the problem of arthritis, and to all other forms of disease, is to know what causes them and thus to be in a position to remove or correct the causative factor.

The truth is that many people, and particularly doctors, are rather reluctant to try to find the causes of disease. This may be because of the necessary change in habits of daily life which might be involved. When people fall ill they do not as a rule ask themselves whether they have been living carelessly and using up their nervous energy, or if they have been eating unwisely and thus piling up troubles for themselves. They want to be cured while still maintaining the *status quo*. They probably fortify themselves with the thought that, while cause and effect may be the logical way of looking at most things, this does not apply to matters of health and disease.

Role of Nutrition

When looking for causative factors in disease we must never overlook the role which nutrition always plays. Nutrition is, of course, the process whereby the nourishment of the system is achieved. It is the fundamental function on which the whole life of the body depends — cells, tissues, structures, the breaking down and building up of the tissues, and the maintenance of heat and energy of the system. The many processes linked with the function of nutrition include mastication, digestion, absorption, assimilation and excretion. Physiologists rightly stress the point so often overlooked — that there are three stages in nutrition: that which takes place in the alimentary tract; that which takes place in the functions of the cells of the system; and that which concerns the organs of excretion. Thus nutrition and elimination are closely linked. We must remember, also, that elimination is not merely a matter of waste evacuated from the bowels — it is a vital function involving the skin, lungs, kidneys and bowels.

Viewed from this standpoint, nutrition is the basic and most fundamental function of the whole system and it plays the major role both in health and disease. Every other function of the body depends upon it. When it is disordered its effect will be felt in every cell of the system. All bodily resistance will be impaired, and in such circumstances anything may happen. Resistance against microbes will fail and the retention of the system's normal waste products (the elimination of which, as we have seen, is largely a part of normal nutrition) will give rise to auto-intoxication with its far-reaching effects upon all the other functions of the body. In particular, it will provide just the kind of internal environment in which the toxins of rheumatism and arthritis can flourish.

It is a mistake to think that food and nutrition mean exactly the same thing. Nutrition is the function of the system that utilizes the food and transforms it into living matter and energy. All-important though this function is, equally so is its dependence upon suitable food to achieve this end. Without suitable food there can be no normal function of nutrition. Development of disease is inevitable where health maintenance breaks down because of this deficiency.

Suitable Food

In all disease, and especially in the form we are now discussing, the question of suitable food is paramount. We are to a great extent, physically at least, the end-product of food that has been utilized by the process of nutrition. Our food must therefore be of the best quality and the proper quantity if we are to be normal healthy human beings. We get our food primarily from the vegetable kingdom. That which we use as animal products derives originally from plants, and plants as living entities derive from the soil and the energy of the sun. Plants, indeed, are the only things which can build up living tissues, and man and animals are solely dependent upon the vegetable kingdom for their food supply.

The human diet is therefore built up from vegetable foods which as we have seen, are the agents which operate between the soil and the sun and develop for us the essentials for human nutrition: proteins, carbohydrates, fats, mineral salts, vitamins and probably many more essential substances not yet known to science. It is as well to remind ourselves that scientists once thought that food consisted merely of proteins, carbohydrates and fats; only quite recently were mineral salts and vitamins given their proper importance in food analysis.

The basic principle we wish to establish here is that the food most suitable for adequate human nutrition is that which is still in its whole state as organized in nature. We depart from this axiom at our peril. Regrettably, today in most civilized countries under the influence of commercial motives, consumer persuaders, methods for preservation and so on, we are reducing human subsistence on fresh natural foods to an absolute minimum. More and more food is becoming increasingly synthetic, and, in losing its freshness in this way, there is no doubt that it is losing also its health-promoting influences. A lesson lies in the fact that in such countries the number of people suffering from arthritis and allied diseases is increasing alarmingly. Indeed, it has recently been pointed out that more than fifty per cent of people past middle life suffer in this way. It is practically certain that environmental factors are the main causative factors, of which food is the most important.

Whole, Balanced Diet

To achieve normal nutrition — and without it no disease process can be overcome — we must include in our diet fresh natural food which is as nearly as possible in the state which nature intended. We must remember that it is through normal nutrition that food bestows its benefits upon the body. Just as we need whole foods for their natural integrity, so too do we need a whole diet for proper nutrition. We need balance between all the foods, for without that balance nutrition will suffer. And here we may say that the division of foods into their various parts, such as protein, carbohydrate, fats, mineral salts and vitamins, has had dangers as well as blessings. For it has persuaded many people that one part of food may be more valuable than another. This has led to the use of an unbalanced diet, particularly in cases of chronic ailments such as arthritis. Another fallacy which has developed in this way is the idea that foods have some special curative value, especially the mineral salts and vitamins. As a result many people dose themselves with these food elements in much the same way as they do with various drugs — and with the likelihood of similarly indifferent results. With the production of some synthetic 'vitamins', the practice is likely to bring much disappointment in its train.

There is no more likelihood of curing arthritis with specific food elements than there is with specific drugs. Incidentally the various drugs now being so commonly employed for all kinds of complaints may well be a real factor in the production of arthritis. It has been established that certain of the powerful drugs produce symptoms which closely simulate various forms of the disease and the fact is now becoming quite clear that drugs of all kinds play a prominent part in the making of this and other chronic diseases. Certainly it is rare to find a case of arthritis where free use has not been made of drugs in one form or another for various complaints. When one remembers the numerous drugs being taken for minor troubles such as constipation, headaches, coughs, colds and so on, and when one bears in mind that these are all foreign substances with no rightful part to play in the nutrition of the system, it is unlikely that we can exempt them completely from blame in the making not only of arthritis but of many other chronic illnesses as well.

Habits that Build Disease

We should remember that many forms of disease are built by daily habits. Taking drugs is only one of them. Smoking and excessive stimulation are others. Mistaken habits of eating — unnecessary snacks when the system is exhausted, bolting food, trying to subsist on prepacked foods and the refined white flour and white sugar preparations — will also lead to faulty nutrition and ill-health. Nervous and emotional habits leading on to mental and physical tensions no doubt play a large part in the making of ill-health. All such habits impose stress upon the bodily organism, and stress leads to enervation. This reduction of nerve force directly affects our nutrition, interfering with the process of elimination by which the normal balance of the system is maintained.

When health and resistance are reduced in this way the

normal wastes of cell activity are not properly excreted and their retention in the fluids and tissues of the body will lead to changes and disease-reactions. From this viewpoint a disease-reaction is not in itself detrimental to the system, and if managed in its acute or early stage along proper lines it helps to restore the normal balance. It is when such a condition is mismanaged by the use of drugs which divert the body's energy, or when the habits causing the trouble are continued, that the body fails to adjust itself. It is when this self-adjusting mechanism has been pushed beyond its limit that chronic disease develops. This is the background out of which such forms of disease as arthritis can arise.

The reason why people differ in their disease-reactions, although the causative factors may be similar, is that the predisposition of the individual determines the nature of the disease that will develop. This predisposition may often run in families and that is why we find many members of a certain family exhibiting arthritic tendencies. Where this does occur there is a real need for the dietetic and other environmental habits of the family to be radically changed if the individual members are to escape the trouble.

While there is no doubt that much can be done to make recovery from the disease complete, providing it is caught in the early stages, the only rational answer to the trouble lies in prevention. From the Nature Cure viewpoint, which we are enunciating, this means taking into consideration the factors we have outlined in this introduction and inculcating them into a philosophy that will govern our way of life — with special reference to the importance of sound nutrition as the indispensable basis of physical and mental well-being.

I.
The Causes of Arthritis

WHENEVER WE THINK of a disease process we should ask ourselves the important question: what causes it? As a rule people tend to think that there must always be a specific cause for each disease; but this belief leads to much misunderstanding. There are few diseases indeed where one factor is the sole cause — because nothing in life is isolated in that way. The same applies to arthritis. There is no doubt that it is allied to a multiplicity of causes and that is why no specific remedy has ever been found to eradicate it. If we are seeking causes then the most rational approach is to examine the habits which characterize the individual's life; we are thus brought up against such matters as eating, drinking, smoking, and the nervous and emotional habits — all the things which make up one's daily routine.

A particular habit does not produce the same reaction in each person. This is because, just as no two peas in a pod are alike, no two humans will ever produce a completely identical reaction. In other words people react in their own and different ways to doses of medicine, particular kinds of food, and heat or cold, stress or strain. Basically this fact is the reason for the different forms of disease which we encounter. A like truth is that the difference in reaction is always dependent upon the idiosyncrasy of the particular patient.

Individual Reactions

This brings us to the problem of predisposition or the diathesis of the patient. In the older textbooks of medicine this term was used much more frequently than it is today and more attention was given to individual reactions. With the development of the powerful drugs there has come a tendency to ignore the constitutional predisposition of the individual. Even so, it is likely that in future we shall hear more about it, because it is in many cases the determining factor which produces the unpredictable reactions to the various powerful drugs about which there is so much alarm today.

Those who develop arthritis have within themselves the seeds of its development. Given an environment favourable to them, these seeds will grow and flourish. Many people think that almost all diseases are caused by microbes and even conditions like rheumatism and arthritis are thought by some to be brought about in this way. True, there are some forms of arthritis that seem to be linked with germ activity, but here again we must remember that these agents become active when environmental factors favour their development, and it is when the normal resistance of the system has changed and deteriorated that such activity occurs. At one time this theory of infection led to much unnecessary surgery. Many a set of teeth has been removed under the impression that in some way they were the cause of the infection which spread to the joints. The same was true of tonsils — often removed because of the same belief — but happily these practices have now been outmoded. What was widely overlooked was that the same factors which produced the infected teeth and swollen tonsils also produced the arthritis.

Peril of Refined Foods

Many of these troubles were the direct outcome of faulty nutrition — i.e., the body had been supplied with foods which rendered normal nourishment impossible. For years now certain foodstuffs have undermined general bodily health and made the development of diseases like arthritis not only possible but inevitable for the person consuming such foods. Nature Cure has, of course, in and out of season warned of the perils of refined, extracted food items like white flour and white sugar and the preparations, all containing a large proportion of these health-destroying articles, which flood the food market. But for some reason the medical profession turns a blind eye on these dietetic dangers and their potency in causing disease. For example, although such foods undermine the nation's dental health, no end of money and effort will be spent in trying to persuade people to fluoridate the drinking water rather than to face up to the true facts of the situation.

And if — as is the case — it has been clearly shown that these foods do undermine the health of the teeth, then it follows logically that their consumption plays a vital part in creating the all-prevalent diseases, rheumatism and arthritis. Experience of these cases has shown that dental trouble in early life is a fairly common accompaniment of arthritis. A study of this aspect of the disease more closely would be worthwhile research. Indeed, when we are searching for the causes of arthritis we must take into consideration, not merely the recent happenings in the patient's life, but the whole case history. There are so many factors that could contribute to the development of such a disease in later life — not excepting the medical treatment meted out in the days of early sickness. It is also worth surveying the long-term effects of the various forms of vaccination and innoculation and their relationship with the development of the degenerative diseases of later life: it is generally accepted that there are long-term as well as short-term effects of such procedures, although at present they are little recognized and understood.

Non-elimination of Body Wastes

Like Rome, disease was not built in a day; and this is especially true of the arthritic complaints. In infancy, as we know, disease reactions are sudden and acute, and with proper management the system is quickly restored to its normal state and function. But with the chronic complaints of later life, the picture is very different. The disease processes persist, and, as in the case of arthritis, changes take place in the tissues and structures of the body. What is clear is that in the acute diseases the toxins developed in disease are quickly burnt up and eliminated, whereas in the chronic forms the elimination of toxins and waste products has been slowed down. When we talk about elimination we must not conclude that this concerns the evacuation of waste matters from the bowels only: all the body's cells, because of their activity, are constantly producing waste products, and these are the vital wastes which may be retained within the tissues and which do the damage. It is at the line of demarcation between the nourishment of the cell and the excretion of its wastes that elimination is so vital to the well-being of the whole system.

Such elimination is directly linked to bodily nutrition. Many people feel that if they have supplied the body with enough roughage in their food it will take care of elimination so far as nutrition is concerned; but this is not truly the case. It has been generally proved that even if there is some slowness on the part of the bowel in evacuating its poisons the system will not suffer directly, and because of this finding it has been argued that auto-intoxication or self-poisoning is a mythical conception of disease causation. But the answer to this is that it is the cell wastes within the tissues that are the real cause of auto-intoxication which is to be found in the fluids surrounding the cells, and, later, in the lymph and the blood.

Intercellular Fluid

When we are looking for causative factors and the part which auto-intoxication may play as the major factor in the onset of arthritis we must think in terms of the life and activity of all the cells of the body, since in the last analysis that is where the initial breakdown occurs. The cells of the body are bathed in a fluid known as the intercellular fluid. This fluid amounts to as much as three-and-a-half times as great a volume as the whole of the blood. In chemical make-up it strongly resembles sea water — which is why it has been remarked that cells live in sea water. There is a constant movement of the intercellular fluid — not a circulation, but a kind of ebb and flow. This fluid is in intimate relationship with the cells and it is in this medium that true assimilation and elimination takes place. Here the exchange is made of the nourishment to the cells and the waste from them. One might say that as long as there is a balanced exchange and free movement of this vital fluid, the function is normal and the individual has good health.

Unfavourable conditions from which the body may suffer are at first experienced in this fluid. First of all its chemical make-up may be changed by the intake of food and drink, and the respiratory function of oxygenation may also be interfered with. When digestion is forced beyond its normal capacity the effects may be felt in the intercellular fluid, and as it is between the fluid and the cells that real assimilation takes place, it is here that the troubles will begin. With the fluid over-loaded in this way the normal elimination of waste products will be impeded and these factors will cause a slowing-up of the fluid movement. And when this fluid is arrested in this way, no matter in what part of the body it may be, we have the congested state which is the first stage of disease, no matter what name we may give to it.

The adverse effects on the intercellular fluids are largely the results of imperfect nutrition. This starts from the stomach and the intestinal tract. When the body is supplied with excess of food, with wrong foods and with all the harmful substances that are taken into the alimentary tract, toxic substances are created which find their way into the tissue spaces to set up congestion and disease processes. Here, then, we have the beginning of auto-intoxication, where the vital intercellular fluid is surfeited with food material and encumbered with cell waste.

Signs of Auto-intoxication

It is out of this condition that a disease like arthritis arises. In a sense the body is poisoned by its own excretions; they are accumulating faster than they are being expelled. While a certain amount of waste products are the normal results of metabolism, when retained in excess over a prolonged period they upset the acid-alkali balance of the system and then it begins to show signs that not all is well within the body. The individual will have a coated tongue, the breath may be unpleasant, there will be a disposition to frequent colds, and the skin will not be as clear and supple as it should be. The eyes lose their lustre and the hair may be dry and lifeless, and nervous irritability may show itself. These are the early signs of auto-intoxication that are never taken sufficiently seriously. Too often they are treated as common ailments requiring only some kind of headache powder, cough cure or suchlike, whereas they really call for a thorough investigation of one's whole way of living, with special stress laid upon the need for better food and nutrition.

If they are neglected and nothing is done radically to change the condition of the system, the disease processes will pass on into the more chronic forms. It is in this state of affairs that the first sign of rheumatism makes itself felt — especially, of course, if the patient has a predisposition to this form of disease. The congestion, having reached what is known as the connective tissue of the body, will cause the various pains in muscles and other structures which may develop into painful bouts of fibrositis and neuritis. There is connective tissue in all parts of the body, so that when it becomes congested the pain can be either localized or widespread. In some cases it is so strictly localized that small painful spots develop, detectable only under pressure.

These spots are often the areas where all kinds of treatments are employed for relief. Hot and cold applications may be used, various forms of massage and manipulation may be applied, and needles are sometimes inserted for the relief which they are said to give. But one should remember that behind all these troubles is the basic operating factor — auto-intoxication — the outcome of faulty nutrition and a reduced supply of nervous energy. Unless this is remembered as the right premise upon which treatment is based, there will be disappointment in the long run.

Disorders of Joints

When this congestion involves the joints and their inner and associated structures, then we enter into what is known as the arthritis field. We should remember in this respect that the word arthritis simply means an inflammation of a joint and when it was originated it was generally thought to be merely a local affair. Today, this view has changed and we now know that arthritis is a constitutional disease. It is, of course, an inflammation of a joint or joints, but that is simply the manifestation of the systemic trouble. The joints are affected in many different ways and its various tissues affected, giving rise to the various terms that are used in diagnosis. In the acute condition there may be synovitis and redness and swelling of the adjacent muscles. The trouble may then develop into various forms. In *arthritis deformans* there may be deformity, overgrowth of bone, loss of movement and wasting of the soft parts. In *rheumatoid arthritis* there may be enlarged cartilaginous development with an involvement of the synovial membranes. *Osteo-arthritis* is said to be primarily an affection of the bony tissues with excrescenses and limitation and complete loss of joint movement. In addition to these forms of the affliction there are some inflammations and disorders of joints directly related to tubercular and similar affections. These, of course, are outside the scope of this discussion.

Danger of Focal Points

Now that we have described many of the causes of arthritis and the way they develop we must turn to another important feature of this complaint. So far we have been concerned with the nutritional and biochemical aspect of the disease, but it is clear that as soon as a joint is involved in disease we must consider the mechanics of the body. Any disorder which affects the structural integrity and mobility of the system must in itself produce certain concomitant factors, and this is particularly true in the case of arthritis. The disturbed mechanics of the body then become inciting causes. In many cases where the affected joints are weight-bearing they are bound to bring about secondary results. When arthritis affects the joints of the lower limbs or of the spine, the whole posture of the body may be disturbed, adding to the difficulties with which the patient has to contend. In addition, the very fact that joints may be under strain may help to localize the disease, so that when the basic causes of the disease are operating in the system it may well be that an injury or a strain may weaken the resistance of a particular joint and become the focal point for the commencement of the arthritis.

This condition is often noticeable after an injury, maybe of a minor character. It may be a strained shoulder, a twisted knee or a similar disability. Where there is no tendency to arthritis and the system is clear of toxic wastes the injury will mend quickly, leaving no trace of the disability. But where there is a tendency to arthritis and the auto-intoxication that precedes it, much more trouble will be experienced. It will take longer to heal and in some cases definite signs of arthritis may be seen. Or, if there is a time lapse between the injury and the development of the later symptoms, the injury may be overlooked and arthritis may be put forward as the primary cause. Careful analysis will often reveal such instances.

The point to be noted here is that such injuries, given the arthritis background, should receive more than the usual care and attention. The constitutional factors involved should be taken into consideration and every effort should be made to improve the general health, paying particular attention to the selection of food and the improvement of nutrition. Much future trouble may be prevented if these important facts are borne in mind. It may well be that the early warning of arthritis will prove a blessing in disguise, enabling one to clear up the underlying trouble before it gets a firm hold on the body.

Handicap of Obesity

Both underweight and overweight people can suffer from arthritis, but as a rule obesity is likely to prove the more serious handicap. The increase in the fat of the body makes the individual more sluggish and interferes with the circulation of all the system's vital fluids, and — as we have already noted — anything which does this tends to set up congestion in which troubles like arthritis can develop. Obesity slows the whole tenor of the system and limits the freedom of the tissues and organs, especially the muscles. As a result, the important organs — heart, lungs, kidneys and so on — are oppressed by the fat accumulation and fail in their function. Such a condition is bound to shorten life and is the medium in which disease will be produced. We cannot say, perhaps, that obesity is a cause of arthritis; we can, however, say that anyone with a tendency to the disease will have his chances of developing it much increased by overweight and the adverse effects which this imposes upon the body.

As we have seen, many factors enter into the making of arthritis, and the idea that we shall one day find a single substance or therapy which will lead to a cure seems quite unreasonable. For the time being, anyway the sufferer is promised very little in that way and it behoves him to adopt methods which have already proved successful in many cases. There is still a great need for everybody to try to understand how much can be done in the treatment of the incurable diseases — so-called — by paying more attention to the *vis medicatrix naturae*, the healing power of nature. But in doing so, of course, it must be understood that each person must take an intelligent interest in the subject and be willing to exercise a good deal of will-power in disciplining himself to make the necessary changes in his or her outlook and habits. From the Nature Cure viewpoint the co-operation of the individual at all times is essential. Also important is the need to start rectifying matters at the first sign of a disease reaction. Taking pain-killers and waiting, wastes precious time. Remember that disease is nothing more than impaired health, and to effect a return to health is the only safe and sane way of meeting the emergency.

From this standpoint the paramount need is to search for the cause of ill-health; waiting for disease to develop and — as in the case of arthritis — cripple the body in the hope that a cure will be found, is a poor line of action at such a time. Cause and effect still operate in the field of health and disease, and we must learn the causes of our disabilities so that we may remove them at our discretion and enjoy freedom from disease.

2.
The Symptoms of Arthritis

TO THE ORDINARY sufferer the word arthritis is in itself discouraging. There is a general feeling that when the arthritic stage has been reached little can be done to eradicate it. This feeling, unfortunately is fostered by the orthodox attitude based upon liberal use of aspirin, since most people know that while this drug may give relief to the painful symptoms, it does not offer anything like a radical cure. Rheumatism, on the other hand, is a word that does not have the same connotation as arthritis; and for some reason people take a rheumatic diagnosis more lightly. But if the fact is borne in mind that there is unity in disease, that one form may easily merge into another, then it is more likely that early treatment will be instituted and consequently be more effective.

People often think that some forms of arthritis are less serious than others, and they console themselves if told that they suffer from *rheumatoid* rather than *osteo-arthritis*. Here again this is the wrong attitude to adopt. It is the departure from health in any shape or form that should be the true criterion and evaluation of a disease, and nothing less than a return to health at the earliest possible moment is the ideal to aim at.

As we have already seen, there are various forms of arthritis. They depend on the constitutional make-up of the individual, but while these variations may interest the research student, they are of little importance to the man in the street. The actual symptoms of arthritic trouble may vary a great deal, from one individual to another, but it may be a good plan to deal briefly with the anatomy and function of the joints so that one may get a better understanding of what is taking place when disease is present.

The many joints in the body all resemble each other in a general way. A joint, or an articulation as anatomists term it, is formed by the union of the ends of bones, and it serves as a rule to provide movement. There are exceptions to this, such as the joints between the bones in the skull, which are immovable. The structure joints may differ somewhat in accordance with their function. Where there is only slight movement, as between the joints of the spinal column, the bony surfaces are united with very strong elastic fibro-cartilages, whereas in the more freely movable joints the surfaces are more completely separated, well covered with cartilage and tied together with strong bands of fibrous tissues, known as ligaments. These joints are partially lined with synovial membrane, the function of which is to secrete a fluid for lubrication of the various parts. The freely movable joints, which generally are the ones most likely to be affected by arthritis, consist therefore of bone, cartilage, fibro-cartilage, ligament and synovial membrane.

We should take special note of the synovial membrane, since this is often the first part of a joint to be affected in disease. It is a thin, delicate, connective tissue and it secretes a thick, viscid glairy fluid resembling the white of an egg. It is a very important tissue in the freely movable joints, investing the inner surfaces and tendons. It is found between surfaces that are interposed on each other and its lubrication is essential to free movement of the parts. It is the tissue involved in inflammation when there is the condition known as synovitis, and it is generally affected in all forms of acute and chronic conditions.

Changes in Joints

We must not think of a joint as being separated from the rest of the organs. All joints are richly supplied with nerves, and with all the vital fluids of the system, and they share in the health and the disease which may affect the body as a whole. We realize this fact in acute illnesses such as influenza or a heavy feverish cold, when the sufferer will complain of aching joints, showing how these are affected in all forms of ill-health. And when the joints are affected directly by disease, as in arthritis, then the symptoms reflect some of the changes which are taking place within them. There will be redness of the skin, swelling around the joint and dull aching pains in the region. These signs are seen in the acute stage when the disease processes are in active progress and when rest is imperative, but later on when the trouble has partially subsided much of the swelling and redness will disappear, although the aching pain may still remain. This is perhaps the crucial time in the arthritic problem: the time when the trouble passes from the acute stage to the chronic because treatment has been ineffective in eradicating the complaint.

If this has happened – and present orthodox treatment makes it most likely – then the stage is set for the slow but irresistible development of the disease. The future symptoms may vary and affect many parts of the body. Then the patient enters the time when aches and pains become a part of his or her daily life. They distribute themselves over many parts of the body – perhaps in the hands and feet with swelling of the joints, amounting to deformity in bad cases. The shoulders, too, may be affected with much consequent pain, especially on movement. Wherever there is a joint we may find signs of the trouble. It may differ in some individuals in the sense that the trouble may be strictly localized in one or more joints; in others, the pains seem to appear at almost any part of the body. When they appear in the chest, as they sometimes do, they may be mistaken for pains emanating from the lungs and heart.

Susceptible Parts

Perhaps because of its weight-bearing functions the hip joint seems to be peculiarly susceptible to the disease. When affected, it proves to be one of the most incapacitating of all arthritic disabilities and is frequently most difficult to eradicate if it has been neglected in the very early stages. It tends to throw the whole locomotor system out of order and produces great strain, especially on the spine. When it is not arrested it may go on to complete loss of function in the joint which alters and impedes the movement of the lower limbs.

The spine is also susceptible to the ravages of arthritis. It is said that X-ray reveals that most people suffer in some way from arthritis of the spine after their middle years — which shows what a hold the disease has on those who live under civilized conditions and with a fast developing synthetic environment. The spine's most important function is its flexibility, and it is true to say that one is as healthy as one's spine. When it is capable of free movement it stimulates the whole circulation, keeps up the tone of the brain and the great nervous system, and promotes the vitality of all the important internal organs. When arthritic troubles develop in the spine, flexibility is quickly lost and the whole body suffers as a result.

'Slipped Disc'

A spine stiffened by arthritis changes in its structure and in its function. The body loses its physical poise, normal weight-bearing becomes a strain and a vicious cycle has begun. Stiffness and a loss of flexibility interfere with the circulation of the spine's tissues and the intervertebral discs suffer in particular. Instead of a free movement bearing evenly upon these structures, they are pressed into positions where the weight-bearing is transferred to the weaker parts and, in time degeneration of the discs takes place. It is from this condition that the so-called slipped disc arises. But discs do not slip. Anatomically it is impossible for them to do so since they are tied with strong ligaments to the vertebra. What really happens is that, deprived of normal circulation and free movement, allied to the fact that they share in the systemic toxic condition, they lose their tissue resistance. When the break-down occurs the discs herniate or rupture — or to put it into colloquial language, they burst. The centre of the disc, or, generally speaking, a small part of it, escapes and if it is in a region where it may cause nerve pressure and irritation, then the excruciating symptoms of the disc lesion occur. In all these cases it is more than likely that there is a close affinity with the rheumatic and arthritic diseases, and this probability is often confirmed by the rheumatic symptoms in other parts of the system which are experienced by these sufferers.

The Arthritic Back

Apart from this particular trouble affecting the spine there is no doubt that among the main causes of backache are arthritis and its allied complaints. In many cases this can be confirmed by X-rays; on the other hand the symptoms may not be developed enough to show on the X-ray and here the complaint may be due to incipient arthritis. In such cases the muscles of the spinal region lose their tone and mobility and the sufferer is unwilling to try to make full use of his back. In time this kind of disability will interfere with the posture of the body, leading to postural strains that will often intensify the effects of the complaints. We again encounter the vicious cycle where the disease produces changes in the body which react again upon bodily efficiency.

Apart from the symptoms already noticed there will be a dull ache in the lower back. This may give rise to more severe crises which may at first be described as lumbago, fibrositis and so on. But if nothing radical is done to clear up the underlying nutritional problems and to restore the mechanical efficiency of the spine it is fairly certain that the more definite forms of arthritis will develop — and, more especially, of course, if there is a family tendency towards the malady.

Another part of the spine frequently affected and leading to symptoms which are sometimes not suspected of having any relationship with rheumatism and arthritis, is in the upper spine and the neck. The neck is subject to much violent action that causes injuries to the spinal tissues and is consequently an arthritic trouble-maker. The neck has to adjust itself in many difficult circumstances. It is often under strain. Jolting in a car, for instance, places a great strain on it and may cause pains to develop in the arms and head later on. If there should be arthritis in the upper spine the condition may become very troublesome. Some forms of headache may be due to these conditions and may easily lead to mistaken methods of treatment. Taking drugs for them is obviously a great mistake and may only postpone effective treatment. These are cases which if neglected in their early stages develop to the point where the uncomfortable neck-supporting collar is the fashionable treatment. The neck structures are particularly vulnerable in the rheumatic and arthritic afflictions; and the recurring stiff neck and creaking joints are early symptoms which should not be neglected.

Those who suffer from rheumatism and arthritis are unduly sensitive to changes in the weather and seem to be able to register oncoming variations with amazing accuracy. Many explanations have been advanced for this phenonemon, but, whatever the explanation, there is no doubt that these 'weather reactors' should take the signs as early warnings of future troubles and should make every endeavour to change their pattern of life and eradicate whatever signs there are of ill-health. Fundamentally the weather probably has little effect in promoting arthritis, providing there is good nutrition and sound health. We should always remember that whenever we react to circumstances in an abnormal way our failure to adapt is largely a question of weakened resistance, and in most cases weakened resistance is a question of inadequate or poor nutrition.

3.
The Treatment of Arthritis

AT THE RISK of reiteration we would say that the most important thing to remember about arthritis is the need to make an early start in adopting effective methods of treatment. Arthritis is, of course, looked upon as a chronic affliction and therefore as fairly hopeless from the start. But this is a misconception which carries the seeds of failure. There is a beginning stage with arthritis, as with most other ailments. In some cases this may be acute and painful; in many others it seems to start off with morning stiffness in various parts of the body, which work off possibly after a bath and the normal activity of the day. The stiffness may clear up for a time and there is a tendency then to think that all is well. But it is fairly certain to return, perhaps in a somewhat more stubborn form, only to clear up again in time.

These recurring attacks go on and in time become more intractable. Often they affect the hands and after a while the stiffness is followed by more acute pain and puffiness. Later, one or more of the joints may begin to swell, presenting us with a definite sign that arthritis is present. By this time the patient may feel that something should be done about his malady and may see his doctor. The diagnosis will, of course, be arthritis. And, unfortunately the stage will now have been reached where the term 'chronic' may be applied and with it the hopeless prognosis of being incurable.

The pain-killing drugs will have helped propel the patient

towards this stage. These drugs (aspirin is perhaps the one most frequently used) while relieving much of the discomfort and pain, will have lulled the individual into a sense of false security. In many ways these drugs do as much harm in postponing effective treatment as they cause in themselves. If taken frequently and in heavy dosage they may cause intestinal bleeding, with anaemia as a possible result; in fact the anaemia so often accompanying arthritis may often be due to the free use of aspirin. The truth is that aspirin has no power to cure the disease; it adds to the toxin content of the system and complicates the issue.

The early signs of arthritis call for urgent treatment, and more especially so if there is a family tendency towards the disease. It may be that no disease is directly inherited but it is certain that where an environment has produced the condition over several generations — as is often the case — we dare not overlook the possibilities of a fertile ground for its development. The urgent need is for a radical change of one's whole mode of living. Dosing with any kind of medicine is not going to bring about this change. What is required is a careful analysis of the daily habits of eating and drinking, together with a properly arranged programme based on a more health-giving plan. In this respect we should emulate the good husbandman who, knowing that poor soil and an unfavourable environment will not produce good results, sets out to improve them. The same fundamental laws apply equally with the human body and the sooner we recognize this fact the sooner will we get rid of the diseases that now plague us.

PART ONE.   DIETETIC TREATMENT

Believing as we do, from long experience in the management of this complaint, that faulty nutrition is a basic factor in the disease and that no certain hope of recovery can be entertained unless the dietetic state of affairs is corrected, we must stress the need for this subject to be given the primary and most conscientious consideration. A radical change in the ordinary diet is urgently called for. In practically all cases of arthritis the diet has been badly balanced, with a predominance of the refined carbohydrate or starchy foods, badly arranged protein and fat foods, and not enough of the essential protective vitamin and mineral salts-carrying foods -- the raw salads and the ripe fruits. Generally there has been added to foods an indiscriminate amount of sugar, salt and other additives which can be harmful in excess.

A fairly drastic preliminary plan is usually needed. It is a good idea to start with a short therapeutic fast which will set in motion the essential eliminative processes; if the sufferer is overweight it will start the reduction that is necessary. If the patient has the will-power, the fasting period should be completed, taking water only in place of any kind of food. If the fasting period is under self-direction it can be carried on quite safely for three days, but if a longer period is needed it must be supervised by someone experienced in the proper procedure. Better still if it can be done in a Nature Cure resort, where there are proper facilities.

In any case fasting is an essential procedure in the early treatment of arthritis, and nothing will clear up the first signs of the trouble more quickly than this self-discipline. Many people shy away from this great curative measure because of popular, and some medical, feeling that it is a mistake to go without food at any time; but this is a mistaken belief. No other measure will provide such speedy relief of the congested state of the inner-cellular fluids which we have already described as the first stage in the development of practically all forms of disease. When the load is taken off the digestive and assimilative processes, movement is restored to the inter-cellular fluid and this stimulates the elimination of the normal wastes of cell activity. Taking the pressure off in this way relieves the symptoms of the disease in all parts of the system.

For this reason the patient will find that abstinence from food will not only quickly reduce the inflammation and swelling of the early stages of arthritis but it will ease the accompanying pains.

One can justifiably reproach the world of medicine for letting this natural and instinctive measure for giving relief fall into disuse. People have tried to substitute drugs because they are easier to use and call for no particular self-discipline and will-power, but there is no comparison between the beneficial effects of fasting and the doubtful suppressive effects of such medicines. Indeed, if ever people are wise enough to abandon the use of drugs, the effects of which are complicating almost every illness bequeathed to the flesh, they will have to return to the simple and efficacious measure of withholding food in times of disease.

How to Fast

Therapeutic fasting is so essential in the early treatment of arthritis that every effort must be made to practice it. Where the patient finds it difficult a graduated plan may be adopted. At first just one meal may be missed; later on, two may be omitted; and then one day of fasting may be possible. Eventually two days and then three days of fasting should be possible. It will be found that most of the difficulties involved are in one's mental approach to the matter; the actual physical and hunger difficulties are practically non-existent.

To modify the fast one can substitute drinks of fruit juices for the water. Any kind of ripe fruit juice may be used but there must be no sweetening of any kind. A glass of the juice may be taken three or four times during the day. It should however be said that the benefits from this plan are not as good as from the straightforward fast; but for all that it is a useful alternative for those who cannot face the complete fast.

When fasting take care to keep warm and comfortable.

Allowing the body to get cold at such a time dissipates energy it can ill afford to lose. It is not necessary to stay in bed but one should avoid extremes of heat and cold at such a time. A reasonably hot bath once a day gives welcome relaxation and is to be recommended, while a full nights' sleep will help to maintain the normal energy of the system. Where there has been a good deal of sluggishness in bowel action it may be a good plan to use a warm-water enema each day during the fast. The aim is not so much to clear the whole colon but to make sure that the lower bowel is emptied. Injection into the bowel of a pint, or a little more, of plain warm water will meet this purpose well and will prevent hardening of any accumulations and consequent pain on passing.

The fasting procedure, which should be instituted at the first sign of arthritis developing, can be repeated at any future time if any of the acute symptoms should reappear. Where the trouble has already developed — and even where joints are affected so that complete recovery cannot be expected — fasting should be carried out to prevent further deterioration. In such cases, to achieve the best results the fasting period will have to be repeated from time to time over some months. It suits many people well to fast for three days every month until satisfactory improvement has been made. Whenever more acute and painful conditions arise they should be met with the fasting period because of its value in reducing the symptoms and giving relief.

Need for Efficient Elimination
The fasting period should be followed by three days on a fruit diet. Any raw ripe fruit may be used and three meals daily should be taken. Fruit food helps elimination not only through the bowels but through the other great depurating organs. It is particularly helpful in eliminating toxins through the kidneys and the urinary tract and during the fruit diet the

amount of urine is generally greatly increased. Sufferers from catarrhal conditions affecting the upper respiratory passages and the chest will find that fruit greatly helps to increase elimination in this respect and in fact offers a permanent plan of correction. In skin complaints – the skin, again, being a most important organ of elimination – the fruit diet is a most helpful aid to recovery. Remember – whatever can be done in a natural way to stimulate elimination will prove beneficial in overcoming arthritis and its allied complaints. Fruit, besides giving excellent results as an eliminating agent, at the same time supplies the body with vitamins and mineral salts in their best possible form and balance.

The fruit diet is also the best one to adopt when the arthritic sufferer is overweight. In spite of all the claims for other preparations offered on the market for weight reduction, there is no doubt that an all-fruit diet will do the work more efficiently and with greater safety. When arthritis is complicated by obesity the patient should stay for a prolonged period on the fruit diet until the body weight is under control. And such a sufferer should be reminded that until the weight has been reduced to near normality, no real relief from arthritis can be expected.

After the three days or so on the fruit diet it is a good plan to omit one meal of fruit and substitute a salad of suitable raw vegetables. The ordinary in-season vegetables should be freely used and, in addition, edible herbs like parsley, mint and dandelion should be included. The salad may be generously dressed with vegetable oil and lemon juice, plus a small amount of salt, preferably sea salt. If salad is preferred to fruit, two meals a day may be taken. In this way the fruit and salad foods should be continued for another three days.

Starvation Diet

The patient may eat quite freely of such foods; these are not items on which people over-eat. Over-eating no doubt is a common mistake behind arthritic complaints but it is generally caused by including in the diet sweetened and spiced-up foods that entice the appetite into excess. The kind of over-eating that is so detrimental in causing arthritic troubles is largely a matter of the refined starchy foods. Cakes, pastries, puddings, sauces, confectionery and so on are the foods responsible for much of present-day over-eating; and it is interesting to note that they constitute a starvation diet, perilously deficient of the most vital food elements, the vitamins and mineral salts. This is the kind of eating from which the arthritis sufferer should divorce himself if he wants to free himself of his infirmities.

Those of us who hold that the only true healing process is the natural function of the body are sometimes accused of using foods as if they were in themselves possessed of curative virtues. It is easy to err in this way, and it has led to many misconceptions about foods and their value in the treatment of ill-health. Many people do in fact speak of foods as if they were healing agents. For instance, honey is said to strengthen the heart, lemon juice will cure such and such an ailment — and so on. The mistake here lies in forgetting that healing is a prerogative of nature and that all that food can do is to build up nutrition so that the system can carry out efficiently its own healing processes. When a person fasts and adopts an eliminative diet the idea is not that these factors do the restoration required but that by using them in an intelligent way we let nature cure. As we have explained, when there is faulty nutrition through wrong feeding, the cells and the surrounding fluid are congested and disease reactions are likely to appear; when we reduce the intake of foods and allow the vital fluids to move and the cells to regain their proper activity health and normality are restored.

The Curative Diet

Fasting and the fruit and salad diet are planned for that purpose. After this course has been followed for the allotted time, we can increase the diet to nearer normality. The fruit and salad diet will constitute the major part of the menu, but we can now add the protein and starchy foods, making the diet complete and well balanced. For example, we may keep to the fruit meal at breakfast time, adding to it, say, wheat germ and milk to make a complete meal. You can of course vary the meal. In hot weather — and for those inclined to be overweight — fruit alone may be taken; if the weather is cold and the patient is on the light side, some wholewheat bread may be added to the meal.

The midday meal may consist of the salad as described; but to it may be added one or more of the starchy foods, such as wholewheat preparations, a little butter, cream cheeses, or potatoes, rice, bananas and so on. This meal, too, may be varied according to the weather and the condition of the patient, remembering that the underweight person can absorb more starchy foods than the one who puts on weight quickly. Such a meal is easily managed from the digestive point of view, so it is probably a good choice for midday, when more work still has to be done. On the other hand, if it fits in better with the patient's plans, the procedure may be varied, the protein meal being taken generally in the evening.

The protein meal might be regarded as the cooked meal of the day. Any kind of lean meat, fish, eggs or cheese can be taken. On the other hand, if a vegetarian diet is favoured, then a suitable substitute must be planned. With this meal two or three well cooked vegetables in season are included — if salad foods are preferred, a well prepared one can always replace the cooked vegetables. The need for cooked vegetables is greater in the winter time when the fresh salad vegetables are more difficult to obtain; so far as food values are concerned, cooking does not increase them, although with potatoes and some other vegetables it adds to their palatibility. And in winter a well made vegetable soup can give good food value and be a very welcome dish.

No one can plan a diet suitable for every individual but the foregoing scheme will provide the basis of one that can be modified to meet special requirements. This régime places more stress upon the importance of fruits, salads and vegetables so that we think of adding the protein and starchy foods and not the other way about – a radical change, since many arthritis sufferers have never given the vital foods – the salads and the fruits – their rightful place in the dietary.

The Normal Diet

A normal diet must be balanced, so that there is a sufficiency of the food elements required for proper nutrition. These must be supplied as nearly as possible in their natural form – the fruits and salads are the ones most easily obtained for this purpose. These foods convey into the system the vitamins and mineral salts, but there is no point in trying to force more of these substances on the system than it needs. Additional vitamins are generally a waste of money – and of vital energy in having to dispose of them. All that are needed can be obtained in the normal food: if there is a deficiency then the diet needs rearranging.

When arranging a normal diet the question of meat must always be considered. If people have no objection to the way it is produced and have no scruples about its use, it can be included as a protein food, and as such will take care of that part of the diet. Even so, it has many disadvantages for the arthritis patient who already has many toxins in the system to deal with. Flesh food is highly putrefactive and there is always the danger of intestinal infection if the greatest care is not taken in its preparation. It is not necessary in the ordinary person's diet and, of the two, the balance is on the side of omitting it from the food of the arthritic. All authorities today, even the most orthodox, agree that a lacto-vegetarian diet is quite satisfactory and there is no doubt that if more people made this their daily choice other vegetable protein foods would be forthcoming that could easily make meat quite unnecessary.

The foregoing dietetic scheme will meet the needs of most arthritis sufferers. Where the trouble has been tackled in the early stages it may only be necessary to go through the scheme once, arriving at the normal diet and then adhering closely to the 'normal' menus we have described. But where the trouble has been suffered over a longer period and where, perhaps, changes in the structures have already taken place, the patient must be prepared to adopt the fasting period several times and persevere likewise with the fruit and salad diet. The scheme works well as a monthly plan, starting with the fasting and following with the special diet until normal diet is reached. Continue until the end of the month and then start the treatment again.

As the condition improves the period between fasting and the stricter diets can be lengthened, readopting the original period only if an emergency should arise. It is not unusual for someone who has made a successful recovery to lapse again into the old nutritional habits, and a watchful eye should be kept for returning symptoms at such times. As we have explained, where there is a tendency to arthritis, disturbances of nutrition are likely to produce the disease-reaction; the patient therefore must always be ready to consider the matter from this angle and ensure that any deficiencies are carefully met. For proper nutrition is undoubtedly the keynote both of prevention and effective treatment. Sir Robert McCarrison's dictum that the greatest single factor in the acquisition and maintenance of good health is perfectly constituted food certainly is true so far as arthritis is concerned.

It is also true that man does not live by diet alone: there are other factors to be considered. As we have said, the body's joints, when involved as in arthritis, provoke problems in relation to the locomotion system, besides calling for relief from the more painful symptoms. There is also the mental attitude to be considered since the general hopelessness that surrounds the problem too often cultivates a feeling of helplessness and despair. And this side of the case we must now consider.

PART TWO.   METHODS FOR RELIEF

The sufferer should still rely on very simple measures for relief of the pain and discomforts which may afflict the arthritic joints. We have already explained how abstinence from food, in acute conditions, will help in this respect, and to supplement this we think that there is no better agent than the use of water. Water is the great solvent and it should be your rule to drink at least two to three glasses daily. And water should be taken in its natural state — tea, coffee and other beverages do not count as water in this respect. Those who find it difficult to drink cold water — and some people do — may use hot water instead. But it should be sipped slowly and no sweetening should be added.

The hot bath is very useful in giving real relief to rheumatic and arthritic ailments. The heat of the bath depends upon the vitality of the patient; if he or she is reasonably strong, it may be fairly hot and prolonged, assuming there are no other contraindications. In a bath of this nature one can relax thoroughly and after a short period thus immersed an attempt should be made to straighten out the limbs and to get a little more movement into a joint where it has been limited. Many find the bath an excellent place to practise joint movement and this should certainly be encouraged. If a pound or so of commercial Epsom salts are added to the bath it seems to make the procedure more effective but this should not be done more than twice a week.

Of course, the effects of the hot bath should be carefully watched. It should never be carried to exhaustion point and one should not remain in it after it has cooled off, making sure not to get chilled afterwards. Remembering these precautions, it should be kept in mind as one of the best ways of restoring movement to limbs and loosening up stiffened muscles. Fifteen or twenty minutes spent in the bath, stretching the limbs and moving the stiffened muscles with the hands, is both good exercise and a good preliminary to a restful night's sleep.

When the joints such as those of the hands and feet are badly affected they should be soaked in a solution of Epsom salts and hot water once or twice a day, in addition to the daily full bath. Use a generous amount of water and when the joints are thoroughly warm try to move and stretch them. The local heat will help to loosen up the joints and soften the tendons and ligaments and often much more movement can be gained in this way without undue pain. If the elbows are affected they, too, may be thus treated; when the hip joint needs extra help one may use a sitting bath with the water just reaching over the pelvic area. If it should be found that the water treatment tends to cause dryness of the skin then a small amount of vegetable oil should be applied after bathing.

When it is not possible to treat a joint in this way because of its position a hot application should be used. Make a solution of hot water with Epsom salts (the quantity is not important — about a dessertspoonful to a quart of water will suffice). This method is sometimes spoken of as the wet pack. Worn linen material such as old sheets are suitable for the purpose. Fold into about four thicknesses and then immerse in water as hot as the hands can bear. Wring out the pack so that it does not drip and then quickly apply it over the part to be treated. Cover it with dry wollen material and leave it on for about an hour.

The hot pack should be used once a day; where there is a good deal of swelling and pain, twice a day will be helpful. In most cases it gives relief from the pain and is a very good way of loosening up the joints, especially if one moves them a little immediately after the application. It is far better to rely on these applications than to fly to the use of drugs which will have no direct effect upon the trouble and only cause toxic complications.

Generally speaking, cold applications are not advisable in arthritic complaints as such sufferers are usually-sensitive to excessive cold and unable to get the necessary reaction from these applications. An exception may sometimes be made, however, when the individual has a 'feeling' for a cold application and enough vitality to obtain a good reaction. In such cases, it should follow the hot pack and the same method should be used, except that the water should be cold, as drawn from the tap.

It is a pity that people do not make more use of the water treatment, not only for relief in rheumatic and arthritic complaints but in many other troubles. So many people are obsessed with the use of drugs for even simple ailments that this valuable measure has been largely overlooked.

PART THREE.   ARTHRITIS AND BODY MECHANICS

We have seen that the basic cause of arthritis lies in faulty nutrition and the toxic state which arises from it. One or more of the joints of the body may be involved and we can understand the whole problem much better if we see how the mechanics of the system are affected and how in turn their disturbed state predisposes to further complications of the trouble. In health our body suffers no undue strain on any of the parts used in locomotion. We stand with good posture, with no strain upon the joints and their structures, and with the body poised so that there is proper room for all the internal organs to function normally. In order that this desirable condition may be fulfilled all the joints of the system must be functioning properly.

Yet even in normal conditions the joints are subject to a certain amount of wear and tear, largely because they have to stand weight-bearing and motion. In good health these functions are carried on normally and the wear and tear is accommodated by the natural adaptative processes of the system. But where there is arthritis the injurious toxins of the disease are carried to the joints and any strain and injuries become complicated by them. The circulation and nutrition of the joints are disturbed and normal restoration is impeded; the tissues around the joint become swollen; and then we have mechanical and chemical irritations to complicate the issue. Like any other machine that is dependent upon mechanical efficiency the impairment of a vital joint in the body will throw the whole mechanism out of order.

This is particularly true, when the disturbance takes place in the joints of the feet, the knees, the hips and the spine. Changes begin to take place in body posture, the flexibility of the spine is lost and this may be followed by interference with the movement of the ribs, leading on to a cramping position of the chest and the abdominal organs. Such a loss of physical efficiency strikes at the very foundation of good health and unless the patient is instructed in methods to prevent further deterioration, the condition will worsen. It is therefore necessary not only to clear up the nutritional and other causative factors which are at work but to restore as far as possible the mechanical efficiency of the whole body.

When arthritis is tackled in the early stages and at a time when it will respond to the nutritional methods we have outlined, it is unlikely that any definite joint disorder will remain, but the patient will be well advised to think in terms of better body mechanics and to institute some corrective exercise for promoting mechanical efficiency of the body. Where there is a tendency to the trouble, any derangement of a joint or joints and any tendency to postural strain must remain a potential danger. In any case, and in the interests of better health and disease resistance, the improvement of body mechanics is a sound investment.

Where the disease has progressed to the point where one or more of the important joints are impaired, then the most strenuous efforts must be made to correct the condition as much as possible and to relieve strain. The most fundamental thing to think about with joint function is that it must be full and free. Anything that interferes with movement, especially in the case of a weight-bearing joint, will upset the balance of the whole body. Restoration of full joint movement, whenever possible, is one of the most important things to be considered in the effective treatment of arthritis.

Restoring Efficiency

We have already said that the hot bath can help to restore joint movement, and the importance of this procedure cannot be over-estimated. One should also bear in mind that movement in a joint can be prohibited for two reasons: (a) if it is going through an acute phase, when rest is clearly indicated, and (b) where there is undue pain on performing the movement. It is clearly necessary when a joint is highly inflamed to place it in the most comfortable position and allow it the maximum rest until the acute condition has subsided. After that a joint should be gently tested for movement, the extent of the movement being governed by the amount of pain experienced. It should only be moved to the point of pain; there is no object in the patient exercising undue fortitude in this respect.

In chronic cases where the joints are more limited in their movement they should all be tested for stiffness and pain. The individual can help himself in this respect, and get some idea of how far the trouble has advanced. Testing a joint simply means trying to find out how much of the full range of movement has been lost and how far the joint can be taken, without pain, beyond the point of stiffness. No undue force should be used; it must be a gentle coaxing movement. Naturally, someone skilled in the manipulation of joints can be of real assistance in such circumstances but forceful movements should never be applied.

Particular attention should be paid to the joints of the spine — and indeed to its whole structure and balance since it plays so important a part in the bodily 'economy'. A simple way of testing the mobility of the spinal joints is to lie on your back on a hard floor and let the curves straighten themselves out. For many people who suffer from the stiff back common to arthritis this may be a trying and uncomfortable position when first attempted. The resistance of the floor will impose a strain on the spine's curves and its rigid areas will not easily give way. Because of the stiffened state of the neck, the top rather than the back of the head will rest on the floor, and the lumbar (low back) curve will remain in its arched position up off the floor.

Corrective Exercise

Rigidity in these regions is potentially dangerous so far as arthritis is concerned. The free-est movement of the spine takes place in the neck and the lower back and when this function is impaired the trouble may settle in these parts and prove very difficult to eradicate. It is wise therefore to try to restore normal movement to these areas. A very thin cushion, placed under the back of the head, helps to straighten out the curve of the neck and stretches the neck muscles and ligaments back into place. If the knees are drawn up, with the feet as close as possible to the buttocks, the lumbar curve is straightened out and it will then come in contact with the floor. While these positions can be used as corrective exercises they are also useful for testing the rigidity, or otherwise, of the spinal area, and in view of their general importance so far as body posture is concerned, they should be practised regularly.

While lying on the floor one may flatten the dorsal (middle) spine by extending the arms above the head. This will raise the chest and expand the ribs; it is helpful while in this position to breathe in deeply so as to take advantage of the extra capacity of the chest. Bring the hands down again and let the chest walls fall as the breath is exhaled. These exercises, practised persistently, will greatly benefit the health and fitness of the body, and will in time greatly improve spinal flexibility which in turn will enhance the efficiency of every joint in the body. For, as the sufferer from an arthritic spine will discover, the spine is the lifeline of the body and its infirmities will make themselves felt in almost every other part.

In many cases of arthritis we find that the joints of the lower limbs, being weight-bearing, are particularly liable to be affected, and they often produce secondary effects upon the body's posture and general mechanical efficiency. When the trouble develops in the feet the effects reflected elsewhere soon become apparent. The arch of the foot has a very important part to play not only in giving support to the whole body, but in helping to balance the body, in assisting to propel it and, to a certain extent, in acting as a shock absorber. When arthritis develops in the feet the arch tends to lose its springlike action and the foot becomes painfully rigid. The elasticity of foot movement is lost, a fact that quickly reveals itself in walking, running and movements of the body generally. It is not an exaggeration to say that if this condition is allowed to go on many other important joints will be placed under strain and the chances of the disease spreading to them quickly will be greatly increased.

The daily hot foot bath should be used, preferably with Epsom salts added to the water, and the arches of the feet should be sprung up and down several times. An attempt should be made, with the feet still in the water, to curl the toes and try to draw them under. This will elevate the arches of the feet and when the grip is released the arches will relax.

This exercise, if performed regularly, will help to restore flexibility to the arches and prevent the arthritis from settling in them.

Knees and Hips
The knees also seem very susceptible to an arthritis attack — possibly because they are weight-bearing and subject to the wear and tear of constant strain. Great care must be taken to make sure that full movement is restored after an attack. During the early stages the hot applications can be used to good effect in treating the knees and they should be continued until the normal function has been recovered. The knees are also subject to injuries, often involving the cartilage, and there is no doubt that if these injuries are not carefully managed and full knee movement restored they may provide a focal point for the development of arthritis. To achieve the return of full movement may need skilful manipulation in some cases.

One should remember that the knee is mostly involved in what one might call a rotation strain, and to strengthen the knee in this respect the deep knee bend is not of much value. The best plan is to place the knee firmly on the floor, about a foot forward, and then use a screwing movement of the leg — first inward and then outward, with the twisting movement centred on the knee joint. Repeat this with the other leg. This movement is not only very useful in helping to restore the strength and function of the knee joint after an attack of arthritis but also invaluable as a follow-up treatment after cartilage trouble.

The hip joint also is frequently involved in arthritis and loss of movement in it will prove incapacitating to the whole body, interfering with many bodily movements and upsetting the balance of the spine. Experience has shown that it is often neglected in the early stages and many people have already lost a certain amount of movement before treatment is commenced. This is a sad mistake because once the trouble settles in this joint it seems to be more difficult to overcome than in any other part of the body. Effective treatment should be therefore instituted at the first sign of the attack, and where there is a rheumatic or arthritic tendency in a family it might be a wise precaution to test the joints occasionally to make sure they are capable of full and free movements.

The hip joint is surrounded by powerful muscles and ligaments and when the joint is affected these structures become tense and unyielding, greatly limiting movement. The hot sitting bath can be of real help in this respect. The patient should sit in hot water deep enough to cover the pelvic area and gently rotate the feet inward and outward, trying to sense a movement at the hip joint. Another useful way of testing and improving the movement at the hip joint is to stand with one foot about twelve inches forward with the weight resting on the heel and the front part of the foot elevated as high as possible. Now rotate the foot inward and outward as far as possible keeping the knee straight and not moving the body. This will affect the muscles and the ligaments around the hip joint.

It should be carefully noted that these joint-testing and correcting movements are not exercises in the ordinary sense. They should always be performed with the idea in mind of gently coaxing the joint back into normal function and at no time should undue force be used; nor should they ever be allowed to cause pain. We have already pointed out that injury to an arthritic joint may make matters worse — and so violence of all kinds, in exercise as well as in ordinary everyday habits, should be avoided as much as possible.

4.
Some General Considerations

THERE ARE SOME general things which the sufferer from arthritis should consider when approaching the matter from the standpoint from which we are discussing the subject. First, there is the widespread and pessimistic attitude towards the complaint which is bound to have some effect on the minds of those who have to face up to the trouble. The general impression is that arthritis is incurable, and many people, once the diagnosis has been made, adopt a defeatist attitude. In this frame of mind it is useless to tackle any kind of task; with so difficult a problem to contend with as arthritis where there is so much need for optimism and a challenging attitude, the defeatist approach is fatal. The struggle has been lost before it has begun.

Defeatism is of course the wrong attitude to adopt towards any kind of illness. It is well known that there have been many cases of recovery from diseases when all the odds seemed to be against it, and there are on record many cases of spontaneous recoveries even from an illness so 'hopeless' as advanced cancer. With arthritis, where there is often a family pattern to guide one, where warning signs of early attacks are clearly marked, and where even in the worst cases the crippling stages are not reached until much time has passed, this pessimistic outlook is not warranted. There is plenty of evidence to show that if the trouble is caught in the early stages it can be cleared and the future safeguarded, and even where the disease has progressed to the stage where some joints have become irrevocably involved, the disease can be arrested and much suffering and discomfort avoided.

Nevertheless, from the ordinary viewpoint there are many factors which tend to develop the 'hopeless' attitude. Much publicity is given to the idea that science is always seeking a cure for the complaint; so it is not unnaturally assumed that if science is still looking for a cure there cannot be much hope for those already afflicted. Reports from research groups propagate the same idea, especially when trying to collect funds for further study. What is overlooked in this kind of publicity is the hopelessness it instills into the patient's mind. Even worse than that, it encourages a wait-and-see, do-nothing -now attitude.

A complete change of outlook is called for. Dr Rasmus Alsaker, who had as much experience as anyone in treating arthritis along rational lines, said: 'If you believe the old fallacy that arthritis is incurable, and give up, you will almost certainly become a prisoner of the disease. But if you tell yourself that you are going to do your best to overcome it, get the correct knowledge, and live that knowledge, you will almost surely recover. A few let the disease become so severe, with completely wrecked joints, that mobility of those joints refuses to return. But even they can generally regain freedom from pain and discomfort. . .'.

Wrong Kind of Attitude

There is no doubt that the proper mental attitude plays a big part in aiding recovery from this complaint. It stands to reason that if one really believes that trying to overcome it is futile there can be very little hope for a successful outcome. Indeed, a defeatist attitude like that will tend to reduce the resistance of the system and make matters worse. Of course, there are some people who are so upset, perhaps, nervously or emotionally, that they suffer their illnesses with a certain degree of satisfaction and, unconsciously of course, refuse to get well. And whenever they adopt a method of treatment they drop it before it has been given a fair trial. Such persons go from doctor to doctor and try one remedy after another.

With the Nature Cure plan, willingness to use one's will power and to be ready to impose on oneself rigid discipline is vitally necessary. This must be clearly understood before a start is made. Unlike medicine, where the patient merely feels that he will get his salvation from taking his prescriptions regularly, the nature curist must realize that he is trying to build and harness the great healing power that is within his own body. To do this takes thought and time and the observance of rules governing the daily habits of life. In short, the patient must be willing to take an intelligent interest in the measures which he has to employ and to be personally responsible for the way in which he carries them out.

While we are discussing the proper attitude to adopt when undertaking treatment, a word might be said about an assumption sometimes held by people who are past middle life. It is not uncommon to hear them say, when they are attacked by a rheumatic ailment or by arthritis, that it is because of their age and that it must be accepted as a penalty of being old. This is, generally speaking, a great mistake. It may be true to say that as age advances the body does not respond quite as well as it did in its earlier years, but it is very wrong to assume that people must suffer because of age. As a matter of fact, if the Nature Cure methods are followed they will have a rejuvenating effect upon the whole system. It is well known that many of the infirmities of advancing age — and, indeed, the ageing process itself — are largely influenced by the retention of the waste products; and anything which assists the natural elimination of these offers the best plan for keeping people healthy and active in their latter years. Therefore, to tackle along Nature Cure lines arthritic troubles in advanced age will not only be helpful in that respect but will add zest and years to life.

Another point to remember when contrasting Nature Cure

treatment with that of medicine is that it is devoid of danger. That is to say, the measures employed will benefit the healthy as well as the afflicted. This fact is particularly true of arthritis. Its treatment cannot be started too early and if one may have been a little premature in adopting such treatment, the gain in general health and toning up of the whole system will have been well worth while anyway. But this sort of reasoning cannot be applied to the taking of medicine.

Nature Cure versus Medicine

Whilst on this point we might well consider the question — What should be the attitude generally adopted towards the use of medicines? The whole idea of Nature Cure is to eliminate from the system the various waste products of the body's building-up and breaking-down processes, and also, of course, the foreign substances that have found their way in as a result of additives in food, preservatives, and so on. It is surely undesirable that further foreign substances should be added by way of medicines. Moreover, medicines, if they have any potency at all, produce reactions in the system and in this way may divert the natural energy which should be dealing with the disease processes. It is understandable that people, conditioned by years of such thinking, feel that no treatment is complete without a medicine. And even if they shun the more powerful drugs, and confine themselves to those whose origins are rooted in folklore, it is being discovered these days that many of the simplest household remedies are not without their dangers. But the real argument against medicines as far as Nature Cure is concerned, is that they are unnecessary. And if you try to get the best of both worlds by mixing medicine with Nature Cure, you will find that medicine inclines the patient along the line of least resistance and thus the exercise of will-power and self-discipline, so essential to intelligent co-operation on the part of the patient, may be lost.

In Nature Cure, health is regarded as the antithesis of disease; therefore everything must be done, not merely to eradicate disease, but to restore health. No matter what form of disease we may encounter we must always remember the general rules and habits which contribute towards the acquisition and maintenance of health. When we consider the best form of diet to adopt for a certain complaint we must watch our eating rules carefully. A well-balanced diet can be spoilt by eating too quickly and not masticating the food, just as we may lose much of its benefits if we eat when we are tired to the point of exhaustion. If there is pain and discomfort in the body, then to eat is usually unwise; you should refrain until normal function has been restored. And as most people are aware when we are under great physical or mental stress, eating at such a time can lead to a badly upset digestion.

The question of physical exercise arises in connection with many forms of ill-health and it is especially important with arthritis and the rheumatic complaints. No one can hope to keep the muscular system in good tone without some exercise; on the other hand exercise is not always easy for those whose work tends to be sedentary and where facilities do not exist for physical recreation. But there is no doubt that we should use the muscles of our body regularly each day, and if this cannot be done by walking or other natural occupation, then some indoor movements may answer the purpose. Gardening is a useful means of exercise, but it tends to be a weekend performance and if the muscles have not been prepared for it, there is the chance of strain, especially to the back.

No Violent Exercise

If arthritis has developed to the point where the joints are affected, then, although exercise is very important, it must always be gentle. Nothing violent should be attempted and the individual should recognize his limitations. An enthusiastic weekend in the garden may put the joints of the back and lower limbs under too much strain and lead to much discomfort. Nor must the sufferer indulge in strenuous weekend games and sport likely to put the joints under strain.

It is extremely important to remember, as we have pointed out, that joint function must be restored by gentle, coaxing movements. This should always be borne in mind by the arthritic sufferer when contemplating exercise. 'Take care of the joints and the muscles will take care of themselves' is not a bad slogan for those who are thus afflicted. It is quite an interesting experience to see how quickly the wasted muscles will regain their shape and tone when freer movement has been restored to the joint whose movements they control. Not even special exercise is needed for this purpose; once the joint is moving freely the muscles quickly return to their normal condition. This is often seen after accidents.

Exercise that brings one into the sunshine and fresh air is very desirable and every advantage should be taken of it. Those who are obliged to live in cities should do their best to get into the country sunshine and fresh air as much as possible, and for this purpose the weekend walk is about as good as anything. But if the sun is at its height in the summer then one must be careful not to overdo it. Sunbathing is of great value for those not allergic to sunshine, but those unable to stand a lot of sun must use great discretion. Exposing the skin to the sun and air will stimulate its activities and prove of real value in arthritis. Such exposure should be done gradually at first; then, as the body becomes accustomed to it, the periods of exposure may be increased. The affected joints may also be treated in this way — with the proviso that over-exposure must be avoided. The sun is a very powerful agent and the source of life and energy, but be careful not to overdo the sunbathing, especially in the early stages.

Air and Friction Baths

An air bath may not be so appealing but from the standpoint of stimulating the skin and promoting circulation it is extremely valuable. Friction applied to the skin of the whole body is a very useful method of toning up the system and there is no doubt that it can be used with real benefit in the treatment of arthritis. Generally speaking, our climate is not conducive to the idea of airing the body in this way, but on the other hand, we should remember that because the climate *is* so unfriendly in this respect, the need for airing the skin becomes more imperative. The skin is not just a covering of the body; it is a vital organ of elimination and its efficient function helps to maintain the health of the entire body. Contact with the air is just as important as cleansing with water.

All these matters are of common interest as far as the health of body and mind are concerned, and they apply to all forms of illness as well as to arthritic complaints. It is a pity that more thought is not directed towards the use of the natural agents, such as exercise, fresh air and sunshine, for the preservation of health and the management of disease, since this would prove the proper antidote to the pill and tablet-taking habit. This obsession with drugs, now fast getting out of hand, may well become a social menace if the present trend continues. Those people who are concerned about it should not forget that the glorification of such drugs started with their use in the treatment of disease. We are reaping the whirlwind of the publicity done for the 'miracle' and 'wonder drugs' so-called — and ordinary people cannot rightly be blamed for thinking that they can solve all their problems — physical, mental and moral — with the drugs which science has provided for them.

Already many people are returning to the idea of whole natural foods; are trying to protest against the inhuman treatment of animals reared for food production; are becoming alive to the dangers for human kind in the use of insecticides and pesticides; and deplore the fast-developing synthetic environment in which livestock is compelled to live. Further progressive thought on these lines should result in the natural agents — exercise, sunshine and fresh air — being used more freely in the treatment of ill-health and the prevention of disease.

Danger of Sagging Bed

Apart from concentrating on our daily activities we should think about the influence upon health and disease of the time we spend at night. About a third of our lives is spent in bed and when a person is suffering from a disease such as arthritis even longer periods may be spent there. The condition of the bed is therefore a matter of great importance and should receive careful consideration. A bed that has been long in use may sag badly in the middle and be a perpetual source of strain to the back. When lying in bed we do not, of course, stay in one position; we are constantly turning about, and if the centre of the bed is not firm the lower part of the back may be subject to severe strain. It is not uncommon for a person to waken in the morning with a strained and aching back due to this strain — a condition that is sometimes the first sign of the so-called 'slipped disc'.

So in order to make the most of a night's sleep and rest we must be quite sure that the bed is firm and gives enough support for the movements of the body. If the bed does sag and for some reason it is not desirable to replace it, then a firm board should be placed under the mattress to provide the necessary support. As a rule, the healthy person requires about eight hours in bed, while one suffering from some disease may need a rather longer period. Generally, those who have a tendency to rheumatism and arthritis should make a practice of getting enough sleep; for nothing reduces the resistance of a sufferer like the breaking of a night's sleep. In many ways sleep is the greatest of all therapeutic agents; it enables natural recuperation to take place and the healing processes go on, using the energy of the body at their disposal.

Learning to Relax

This fact is recognized by doctors, who try to induce sleep in the patient by means of drugs. But sleep produced in this way and natural sleep are by no means the same thing. Much can be done to induce sleep by conscious relaxation of the muscles and when there is difficulty in sleeping this should be practised. It is a good plan to try relaxing the various parts of the body; try first to let the feet relax, then the muscles of the legs and then the muscles of the upper part of the body. It is also helpful to control the breathing thus: breathe in deeply; then hold the breath and count five before exhaling; then breathe in again; hold the breath, count five, and so on. This will often take the mind off prevailing troubles and let the body and mind relax.

Apart from the time spent in bed it is wise to set aside a few minutes each day for the purpose of relaxing the system and relieving some of the tensions. This is mostly a matter of practice. As time goes along and one gets used to shutting off the activities and energy, it will become possible for this to be accomplished in a matter of seconds. Some people can not only shut off in this way but actually fall asleep for a minute or two and awake much refreshed. It is the shutting off process that relieves the tension. All those who suffer from a complaint like arthritis, where so much of their energy is constantly being used in meeting the extra demand of the body, should make a point of learning this kind of relaxation. It is easier to do than to describe, but most people, if they will be patient, can accomplish it for themselves, with real benefit from the point of view of regaining their health.

Résumé

Arthritis, in all its forms, is a constitutional disease, in which the joints of the system are affected. It may be of the acute or chronic kind.

There is often a strong family tendency in which members of various generations may be affected.

The basic cause is auto-intoxication resulting from faulty nutrition. Once this condition is established there may be many inciting causes, including nervous and emotional strains, overwork, and in fact anything which lowers resistance.

Recovery depends upon early treatment; if the disease is allowed to progress, the joints may be involved beyond repair.

Rest inflamed joints; loss of movement in joints should be restored by gentle, coaxing movement; no forcing effort should be used.

Adopt fasting as the important therapeutic measure. Follow instructions.

Follow with fruit and vegetable diet.

Build up a well balanced diet with a generous amount of fresh fruit and raw salads.

Repeat the fasting and the fruit and vegetable diet from time to time as may seem necessary.

Relieve the inflammation and swelling of joints by water treatment. Use hot baths and hot packs for relief and for help in mobilizing the joints.

Make a special effort to limber up the spine and improve the posture.

Adopt proper positions in relation to the weight-bearing joints as in the hips, knees and feet.

Avoid straining the joints and be sure that full movement is restored to a joint after an injury.

Avoid violent exercise.

Adopt health-building measures, get moderate exercise in the open air and sunshine and a full quota of sleep and rest. Learn to relax the muscles of the whole body.

Catch the trouble in the early stages; chronic cases need patience and persistence to achieve worthwhile results.